CAN I TELL
YOU ABOUT
MULTIPLE
SCLEROSIS?

CAN I TELL YOU ABOUT...?

The "Can I tell you about...?" series offers simple introductions to a range of limiting conditions and other issues that affect our lives. Friendly characters invite readers to learn about their experiences, the challenges they face, and how they would like to be helped and supported. These books serve as excellent starting points for family and classroom discussions.

Other subjects covered in the "Can I tell you about...?" series

ADHD	Epilepsy
Adoption	Gender Diversity
Anxiety	ME/Chronic Fatigue
Asperger Syndrome	Syndrome
Asthma	OCD
Autism	Parkinson's Disease
Cerebral Palsy	Pathological Demand
Dementia	Avoidance Syndrome
Depression	Peanut Allergy
Diabetes (Type 1)	Selective Mutism
Down Syndrome	Sensory Processing
Dyslexia	Difficulties
Dyspraxia	Stammering/Stuttering
Eating Disorders	Stroke
Eczema	Tourette Syndrome

CAN I TELL YOU ABOUT MULTIPLE SCLEROSIS?

A guide for friends, family and professionals

ANGELA AMOS
Illustrated by Sophie Wiltshire

Jessica Kingsley *Publishers*
London and Philadelphia

First published in 2017
by Jessica Kingsley Publishers
73 Collier Street
London N1 9BE, UK
and
400 Market Street, Suite 400
Philadelphia, PA 19106, USA

www.jkp.com

Library of Congress Cataloging in Publication Data
Names: Amos, Angela, author. | Wiltshire, Sophie, illustrator.
Title: Can I tell you about multiple sclerosis?
: a guide for friends, family
    and professionals / Angela Amos ; illustrated by Sophie Wiltshire.
Description: London ; Philadelphia : Jessica
Kingsley Publishers, 2017. |
    Includes bibliographical references and index.
Identifiers: LCCN 2016031973 | ISBN 9781785921469 (alk. paper)
Subjects: LCSH: Multiple sclerosis--Juvenile literature.
Classification: LCC RC377 .A566 2017 | DDC 616.8/34--dc23
LC record available at https://lccn.loc.gov/2016031973

British Library Cataloguing in Publication Data
A CIP catalogue record for this book is
available from the British Library

ISBN 978 1 78592 146 9
eISBN 978 1 78450 413 7

Printed and bound in Great Britain

ACKNOWLEDGEMENTS

To my loving family, Alistair, Zoe, Emily and Cathy. To Anthony and all those friends who have helped me along the way. Thank you.

CONTENTS

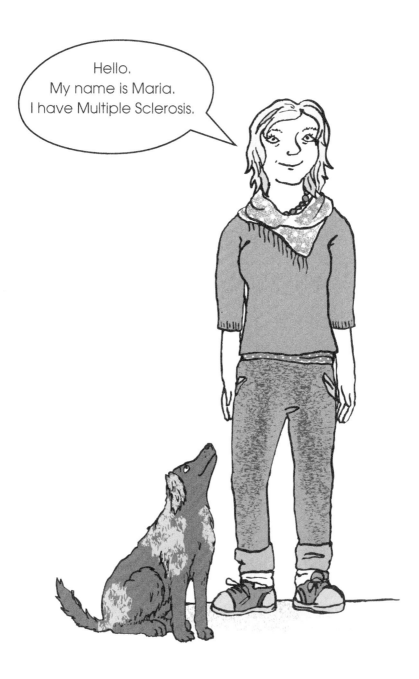

"Last year I found out that I have Multiple Sclerosis or MS for short. Everyone with MS is affected differently but I think that if I tell you about what happened to me it might help you to understand more about it. I hope that reading my story will help you feel less unsure or worried about MS. Then if you meet someone who has MS or if you find that someone in your own family has MS you will know much more about it."

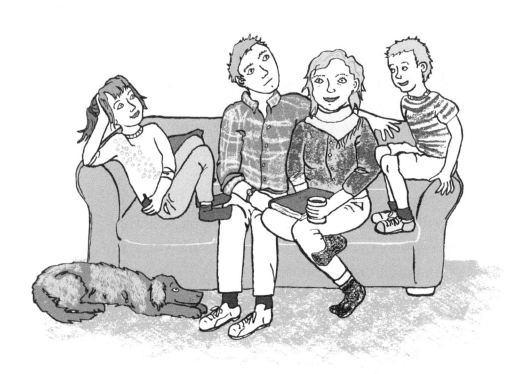

"This is my family – Ben, Cara, Dino
and Teddy our dog."

"Before I tell you any more though, I'd better introduce you to my family. This is Ben, my husband, Cara who is 14 years old, Dino who is 10 years old and our dog, Teddy. We all get on pretty well, most of the time! It helps having Teddy around because if we are feeling upset he loves to look after us!

One of our favourite times is the summer holidays. Cara and Dino are off school and Ben and I take some time off work. Sometimes we stay at home and other times we go away on holiday. We always try to have a fun time, doing things that we can all enjoy together, including Teddy. But last summer felt different..."

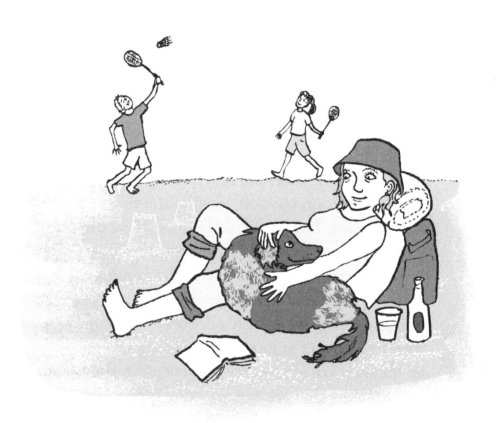

"I had no energy, I had to keep resting. I
started to feel dizzy and felt like I was
moving even when I was sitting still."

"Before we left to go on holiday, I was feeling unwell. I was finding it difficult to remember to pack everything we needed. I felt like a battery that needed to be recharged. Everyone was feeling excited about our holiday but I just felt like lying down. The side of my face and the inside of my mouth became numb. Everyone said that my face looked normal, but I felt like one side of my face was frozen.

Once we were away, my energy seemed to slip away even more. I had to keep resting, I couldn't keep up with the others."

66 **I** started to feel dizzy. Even when I was sitting down safely I felt like I was on the move.

One day my energy disappeared completely. I felt like a balloon that had had all its air let out of it. I had to spend a day resting, and I missed a trip to a chocolate factory, which I had been looking forward to. Cara and Dino went with Ben, and they brought a treat back with them. Chocolate!

Later on when we were home again, I noticed that my feet were very cold. I felt like I had ice blocks for feet even on sunny days! The last thing I remember happening that summer was that my legs became very weak. My legs stopped doing what I expected them to do, like I wasn't able to rely on them anymore. I had to really concentrate on walking, because if I didn't, I fell over.

After talking to my local doctor, Ben took me to hospital."

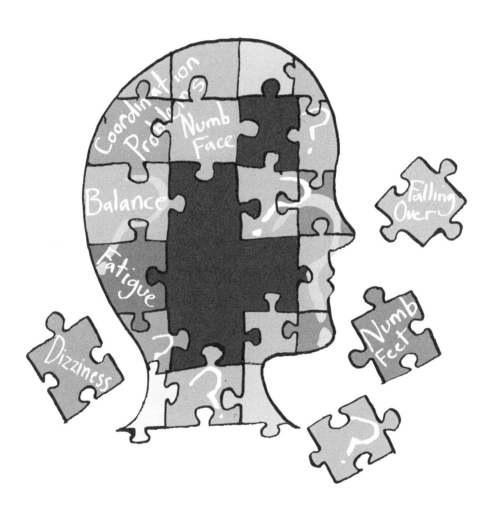

"I had a lot of different symptoms."

"Once at hospital I met some very helpful people. A doctor asked me lots of questions about what was happening now in my body and also helped me remember other changes that had happened before our holiday. The tricky thing about MS is that you can experience a lot of different symptoms, and I had not realised that they were all connected. It felt a little like piecing a jigsaw puzzle together, each symptom being a different piece of the puzzle. I think the doctor had an idea of what my jigsaw picture was starting to look like, but I was still feeling puzzled. The doctor arranged for me to be admitted into hospital, so that I could have some tests."

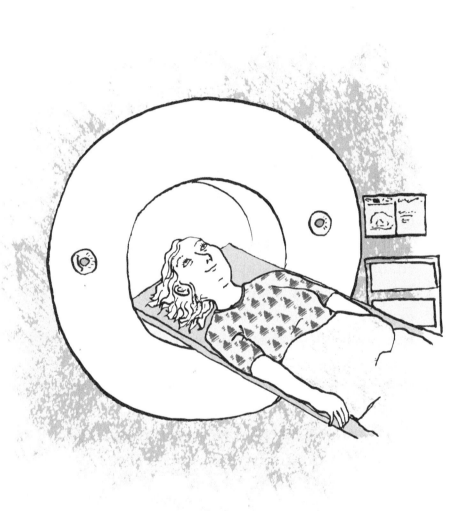

"I had an MRI scan. This took photographs of
my brain and spine. The photographs showed
where the MS was in my brain and spine."

"One of the tests I had was called an MRI scan. MRI is short for Magnetic Resonance Imaging. For this test I had to lie in a special capsule that took clever photographs of my brain and spine. These photographs were very useful because they showed where MS was active and had been active in the past in my brain and in my spine. I'll explain more about that later. So after a few more tests to rule some other diseases out the puzzle was complete. The doctor talked through what they had discovered and then a nurse met with me to talk some more about my diagnosis of MS.

There are different kinds of MS; my diagnosis was active Relapsing Remitting MS. This kind of MS means that some of the time I will experience symptoms; this is called a relapse. Other times I may be free of symptoms; this is called a remission. You can read more about this later. I felt shocked and tearful at first, but I also felt relieved that my puzzle had been solved. The doctor and nurse really understood how I felt and gave me some helpful information to take home with me, so that I could understand more about MS. I was also given some tablets called Steroids to take for five days to help with my current symptoms."

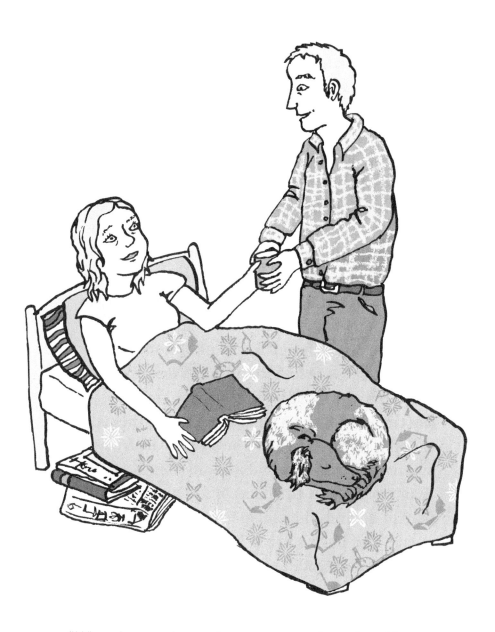

"When I came home I was very weak and walking
felt difficult. Ben made me a bed in our front
room so that I didn't have to climb the stairs."

"It took several months to recover from the relapse. To begin with I felt very weak and walking felt very difficult. I felt like a feather that could be blown away by a puff of wind. Ben made me a bed downstairs, so that I didn't have to climb the stairs. Teddy loved this, because it meant that he got to sleep at the end of my bed; something he is not allowed to do normally! Gradually I started to feel better. I was able to spend less time resting and could move around more. My strength increased, and I was able to walk around using a stick. I started to build up my strength by walking around our garden. It felt so good the first time I felt strong enough to take Teddy for a walk again."

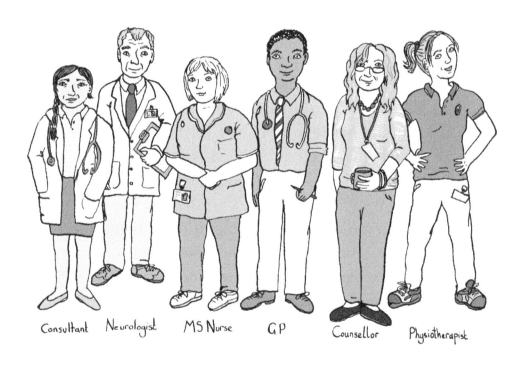

Consultant Neurologist MS Nurse GP Counsellor Physiotherapist

"Once I was diagnosed with MS, I was offered
a lot of professional support. There is a whole
range of professionals who can help."

"It feels good to know that I have people who really understand about MS, who can advise and support me when I need it.

When I was first diagnosed with MS I found it helpful to talk to a counsellor. I was able to share how I was feeling which in time helped me to accept the diagnosis."

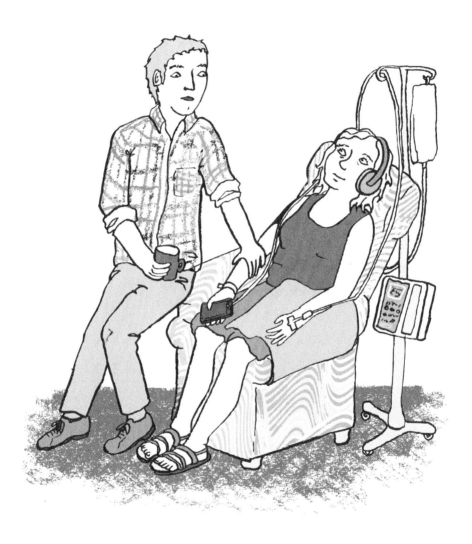

"There are different kinds of treatment for MS and they work in different ways. I go into hospital every month for an infusion."

"There are several different kinds of treatment available for MS, and they work in different ways. These treatments come in tablets, injections or infusions. Not all treatments suit everyone and it took a while to find the best option for me. I go into hospital every four weeks for an infusion. This means that the drug I take comes in a liquid. The medicine moves into my body from a bag, through a tube and into a vein. At first I felt a little scared, but I have got used to it now. I have a comfy seat to lie back on, and I bring my favourite music to listen to while I am having the infusion. There isn't a cure for MS, but the treatment I have helps to reduce the damage to my brain and spine as a result of my having MS."

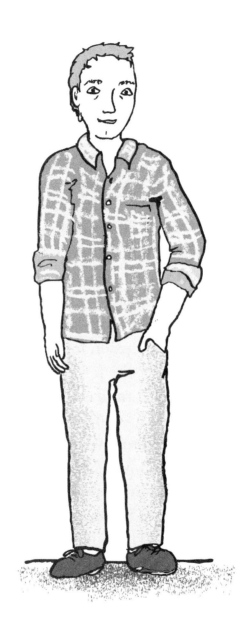

"MS has meant changes for all of us."

66**I** felt shocked when Maria was given her diagnosis. I knew that Maria had been unwell over the summer, but I had thought that she had a virus. I feel bad that I didn't realise what was going on, but know that I couldn't have known really.

When Maria was recovering from her relapse, I needed to take some time off work to help look after her. My manager was very understanding and allowed me to work from home some of the time. Once Maria got a bit stronger, I arranged to pop home at lunchtime to see her before going back to work. We have some good friends who also helped by looking after the children, cooking us meals and just being at the other end of the phone if Maria needed any help. I understand now just how good it is to have friends.

Now that Maria has recovered from the relapse and is able to be more active again, life is easier, but it will never go back to how it was. Maria has had to cut down on the amount of work that she does, because she suffers a lot from fatigue. Maria isn't able to be as active as she used to be. This isn't really a bad thing though – she was a bit of a workaholic! One of the difficult aspects of MS is living with the uncertainty around the disease. Maria has good days when she feels energetic and bad days when she needs to rest more. The problem is we never know how she is going to feel from one day to the next. This makes planning difficult to do.

We also don't know when or whether she is going to have another relapse or how MS may affect her in the future. We hope that the treatment Maria is receiving and the lifestyle changes she has put in place will reduce the likelihood of this happening, but I still have that concern in the back of my mind. Maria says it's about learning to live in the moment more, appreciating the good times, but this is more difficult than it sounds…

I feel really proud of how Maria has coped with her diagnosis. I don't know how I would have reacted if it were me. We are now learning to live in a more relaxed and healthy way, which has got to be good for all of us!"

"When we left to go on holiday, I sensed that Mum wasn't quite her normal self, but I didn't think it was anything to worry about. When Mum first told us that she was feeling ill, I couldn't understand what was wrong. Mum just looked normal. The odd thing was one day Mum seemed to be okay and the next she needed to rest. It stopped us from doing some activities on holiday, which was disappointing.

When Mum got taken into hospital, I was really worried, Mum had never had to stay in hospital before, so I figured it must be serious. When Mum and Dad told us that Mum had MS, they explained the basics to us. Mum showed me a website that one of the nurses had recommended, so that I could find out more information. I was worried about the chances of me getting MS, but I found out that it isn't something Mum can pass on to me. Mum and Dad let our close friends know what was going on. This was really helpful, because it meant that I didn't need to explain it to everyone and friends texted me to see how I was.

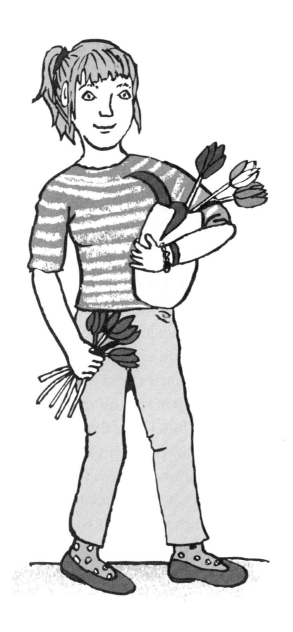

"When Mum is ill, I need to help
around the house more."

When Mum was having her relapse, she wasn't able to move around very easily. Dad set up a room for her downstairs, where she could sleep and rest. We joked that our house had become a florist, because friends and family sent us a constant supply of flowers! I needed to help out a lot more around the house, keeping an eye on Dino and making drinks for Mum when Dad was at work.

Gradually Mum got stronger again, and life seems like it is back to normal. Mum's had to cut down on how much work she does, so we don't have so much money, though this does mean that Mum is around a lot more for a chat after school. I think Teddy has really enjoyed having Mum around more at home. He loves having Mum for company."

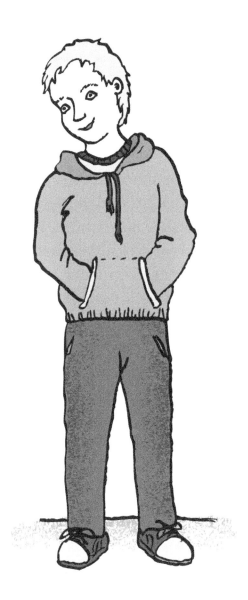

"We have had to get used to changing our plans."

"When Mum came out of hospital, I was really worried. She was very pale and weak. Once Mum and Dad explained about MS, though, I felt relieved. I was scared Mum was going to die, but Mum explained that MS is a condition that she will always have and that she will learn to manage it. It felt sad when Mum was having the relapse, because it stopped her from joining in. Mum couldn't make my birthday party that year, but I told her all about it when I got home. Mum spoke to my teacher at school and told her what had happened. My teacher told me that I could come and talk to her if ever I needed too. Mum and Dad also let my best friends know. It turns out that my friend's Grandma has MS so he really understood."

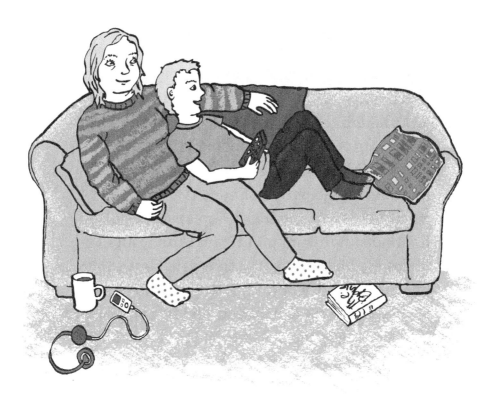

"At first I felt cross that Mum needed to rest a lot more but now I am enjoying the rest times too!"

"Now that Mum has recovered from the relapse she is able to do a lot more. Sometimes, though, we have to change our plans because Mum feels too tired, and this can feel really disappointing. I felt quite angry about this at first, because when I feel tired, I still have to do things! Mum explained that when she is very tired, it is because she is suffering with fatigue. Fatigue is different from feeling tired and can affect Mum in different ways. Mum describes it as one of her 'foggy days', because it feels a bit like walking through thick fog. On these days Mum's thinking is slower, and she finds it harder to remember and say the right words. Mum's legs can feel spongy and weaker than usual, and her balance may not be so good. On foggy days Mum's energy is lower than normal too. At first I was worried that it was my fault that Mum was so tired, but I know now that it's her MS. Mum is learning to cope with her foggy days and finds that having rest times each day really helps. I've started to enjoy these rest times too!"

"I have had to make quite a lot of changes in my life since my diagnosis. It feels a bit like when you buy a cake that turns out to be a lot smaller than you imagined: for everyone to get an equal slice, it needs to be cut carefully. My day has to be divided carefully, so that I can manage it as best I can. I have to decide on which activities are most important and which can be put off for another day. I have reduced the amount of hours I work, so that I have time to rest to recharge my batteries before Cara and Dino return home. If I have had a very busy day, I try to make sure that the next day is easier. I have learnt to take each day as it comes. When I am feeling good, I do more, and when I don't, I do less. I can feel frustrated, but I have really had to learn to listen to myself and how I am feeling and not give myself too much of a hard time when I am feeling less well."

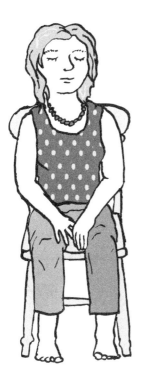

"Over time I have discovered things that help me manage my MS.

Mindful Meditation helps me to enjoy the present moment more and worry less about the future.

Shiatsu Massage helps to relieve bodily tension and helps me relax.

Qigong helps me to feel relaxed and strengthens my balance.

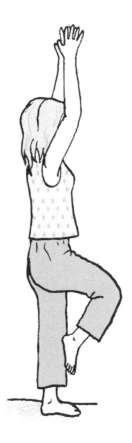

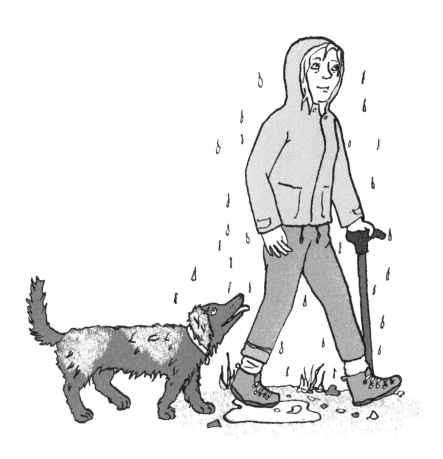

Walking Teddy helps both of us feel good!

Eating a healthy diet.

Medication that works well for me.

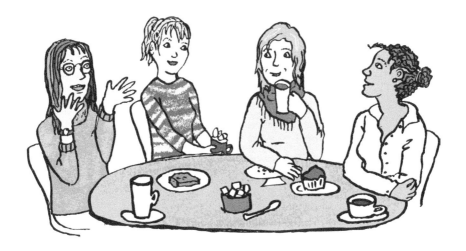

Support from friends and family.

Rest and relaxation.

Over time I have learnt to accept that I have MS. It has helped me to remember that I am still just Maria and that MS is only part of me."

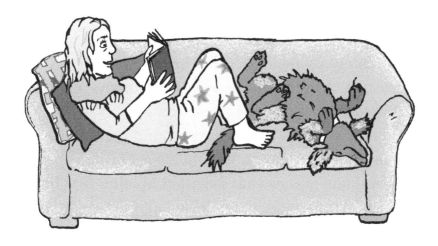

WHAT IS MS?

We have a very clever system inside us that helps our bodies do what we want it to do. We have nerves in our brain and spinal cord. These nerves send messages to and from the brain, travelling along our spinal cord to different parts of our body. For example, if you are walking to school and notice a friend ahead, your brain will send a message to the muscles in your legs, so that you can start to run to catch up with them. Messages are being sent all the time around our bodies. Right now my brain has been sent a message to tell me I have an itch on my head, and my brain has sent a message to my hand instructing it to give my head a scratch!

The messages that whizz around our bodies have to move quickly. We have a covering around our nerves that is called Myelin. Myelin acts as a protective coat for our nerves and also helps the messages travel fast.

We all have an immune system, which is made up of cells in our body that help protect us from germs that can be harmful to us. It is our immune system that helps us recover from coughs or colds or helps us not even catch them in the first place. However, when someone has MS, their immune system is in a state of confusion. Their immune cells think that the Myelin that protects the nerves shouldn't be there and is harmful. This is a problem, because the immune cells attack the Myelin and, in trying to get rid of it, damage it. When the Myelin is damaged, messages can't get sent as quickly or can't get through at all. The kind of difficulties a person with MS has will depend on where the Myelin has been damaged. Sometimes the body is able to repair damage to the Myelin. This is why some MS symptoms can improve over time and others remain a problem.

DIFFERENT KINDS OF MS

There are different kinds of MS.

RELAPSING REMITTING MS

With this type of MS, the person has symptoms
for a period of time. This is called a relapse.
A relapse can last anywhere from two days
to many months and can vary in severity.
People have several relapses in a year or can
go several years without having a relapse. A
person can recover fully or partially from a
relapse. Times when a person is symptom free
are called remission.

PROGRESSIVE MS

This is when symptoms become worse
gradually over time. The speed at which this
happens varies and can't be predicted.

There are two kinds of Progressive MS:

SECONDARY PROGRESSIVE MS

Sometimes, over the years, a person with Relapsing Remitting MS finds it harder to recover from relapses and their symptoms get gradually worse. They find that they have increasing disability. This is called Secondary Progressive MS.

PRIMARY PROGRESSIVE MS

This is a kind of MS where a person's symptoms of MS get steadily worse from the beginning rather than having relapses and remissions.

BENIGN MS

This is when someone has had very mild symptoms with very long periods of having no symptoms. Normally a person has to have been free of symptoms for at least ten years before receiving this diagnosis.

RECOMMENDED READING, WEBSITES AND ORGANISATIONS

BOOKS FOR CHILDREN AND YOUNG PEOPLE

Multiple Sclerosis Trust (2009) *Kid's Guide to MS*. Letchworth Garden City: Multiple Sclerosis Trust.

Mutch, K. and Whittam, A. (2010) *The Young Person's Guide to MS*. Letchworth Garden City: Multiple Sclerosis Trust.

BOOKS FOR ADULTS, FAMILY MEMBERS, FRIENDS AND PROFESSIONALS

Jelinek, G. (2016) *Overcoming Multiple Sclerosis*. London: Allen and Unwin.

Kabat-Zinn, J. (1996) *Full Catastrophe Living: How to Cope with Stress, Pain and Illness using Mindfulness Meditation*. London: Piatkus Books Ltd.

Mills, N. (2010) *Qigong for Multiple Sclerosis: Finding your Feet Again*. London: Singing Dragon.

WEBSITES

UK

Headspace

www.getsomeheadspace.com

Multiple Sclerosis Society

www.mssociety.org.uk

Multiple Sclerosis Trust

www.mstrust.org.uk

The North Wales Centre for Mindfulness Research and Practice

www.bangor.ac.uk/mindfulness

AUSTRALIA

MS Australia

www.msaustralia.org.au

USA

Multiple Sclerosis Association of America: MSAA

www.mymsaa.org

WORLDWIDE

Overcoming Multiple Sclerosis

www.overcomingms.org

ORGANISATIONS

BACP – British Association for Counsellors & Psychotherapists

1 Regent Place

Rugby

CV21 2PJ

Phone: 0870 443 5252

Website: www.bacp.co.uk

OMS – Overcoming Multiple Sclerosis
Thame House
Thame Road
Haddenham
Bucks
HP17 8HU
Website: https://overcomingms.org

Multiple Sclerosis Trust
Spirella Building
Letchworth Garden City
Hertfordshire SG6 4ET
Phone: 08000 323839/01462 476700
Email: info@mstrust.org.uk
Website: www.mstrust.org.uk

MS Society
372 Edgware Road
London
NW2 6ND
Phone: 0208 428 0700
Website: www.mssociety.org.uk

Shiatsu Society
PO Box 4580
Rugby
Warwickshire
CV21 9EL
Phone: 01788 547900
Website: www.shiatsusociety.org

CAN I TELL
YOU ABOUT
MULTIPLE
SCLEROSIS?

CPI Antony Rowe
Eastbourne, UK
June 20, 2023